Sleeping Bag Yoga

STRETCH! RELAX! ENERGIZE!
FOR HIKERS, BIKERS & KAYAKERS

UPDATED EDITION

Erin Widman

illustrations by Jean Bradbury

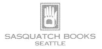

SASQUATCH BOOKS
SEATTLE

Thanks to all the teachers who have taught me so much, especially Denise Benitez, Ulla Lundgren, Noah Maze, and John Friend. Thanks to Bob Hoffa for his assistance. My deepest gratitude and appreciation goes to my loving family, Andy, Noah, and Ruby Bessler, for it is their presence in my life that is the greatest gift.

Copyright © 1999, 2008 by Erin Widman
Illustrations copyright © 2008 by Jean Bradbury

Printed in Singapore by Star Standard Industries Pte Ltd
Published by Sasquatch Books
Distributed by PGW/Perseus
15 14 13 12 11 10 09 08   10 9 8 7 6 5 4 3 2 1

Cover and interior illustrations: Jean Bradbury
Cover design: Lesley Feldman
Interior design: Lesley Feldman
Interior composition: Liza Brice-Dahmen & Rosebud Eustace

Library of Congress Cataloging-in-Publication Data
Widman, Erin
   Sleeping bag yoga : stretch! relax! energize! for hikers, bikers & kayakers / Erin Widman ; illustrations by Jean Bradbury.—Updated ed.
        p. cm.
   Previous ed.: 1999.
   ISBN-13: 978-1-57061-554-2
   ISBN-10: 1-57061-554-3
   1. Hatha yoga. 2. Outdoor life–Health aspects. 3. Sleeping bags. 4. Tents. I. Title.

RA781.7.W536 2008
613.7'046–dc22

                              2007044498

Sasquatch Books
119 South Main Street, Suite 400
Seattle, WA 98104
(206) 467-4300
www.sasquatchbooks.com
custserv@sasquatchbooks.com

·· contents ··

·• introduction •·

I was two months into the excursion of a lifetime: bicycle touring, backpacking, and kayaking in New Zealand and Asia. Having just completed a leg of high-mountain trekking, I was returning to my main mode of transportation: cycling. I was in the best physical and mental shape of my life, yet the prospect of pedaling up mountainous roads seemed daunting. A chronic tightness in my neck was leaving my spirits dragging. Unless something changed, I didn't see how I could complete my travels—let alone enjoy myself.

During one of those inevitable moments of longing for the comforts of home, I realized what was missing. I was pushing my capabilities to the limit on this demanding trip without paying any attention to my body's subtle needs. Back in Seattle, I was typically on my yoga mat every day, tending to my physical and mental well-being. On this trip, I hadn't practiced once. With all the new places to explore and the challenges of pedaling, hiking, and paddling, I simply had not given myself time.

One morning, as I was considering easing my stiff body out of the tent, it occurred to me that my sleeping pad and bag were roughly the same size as my yoga mat back home,

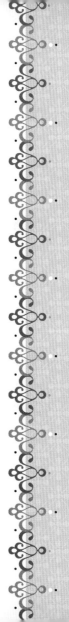

and that they could serve the same purpose. Turning over in my sleeping bag, I pushed up into a position called "downward facing dog." Replaying the quiet voice of my yoga instructor while stretching my back was exactly what I needed.

During the rest of my trip, I developed a series of yoga positions that could be executed in a limited space—inside my small backpacking tent, either in or on top of my sleeping bag. From the broad array of yoga positions, I was able to select those that stretched, relaxed, and energized the specific muscles that had tightened during a strenuous day of hiking, cycling, or paddling. Soon the tightness in my neck disappeared and I succeeded in reaching my destinations with body relaxed and spirit soaring.

You don't have to be an extreme-sports enthusiast to derive benefits from *Sleeping Bag Yoga,* nor do you need any previous yoga experience. These positions have been culled from a wide range of possibilities, with simplicity and safety in mind. If you kayak and beach camp for a few days, your upper body will get a workout as your lower body stiffens in the tight compartment of your boat. Stretching at the end of the day will be soothing and relaxing. A routine in the morning will revitalize you for another day of paddling so you can continue your adventure in the spirit of play. Yoga can confer similar benefits when you're hiking—whether it's months on the Pacific Crest Trail or even a day hike in the Olympic Mountains. *Yoga* literally means "to yoke" or "union." Therefore any moment in which we are strong in our body and in tune with our surroundings, we are linked into all that yoga has to offer.

While geared to enhance the capabilities of the body in sport, the yoga positions presented here also encourage alignment and harmony with nature. They draw upon and express a yogic philosophy that all of nature, including our bodies, is simply an expression of a divine spirit at play, that life is a gift to be received. This view confirms what hikers, bikers, and paddlers already know; we act from this perspective every time we set out on an excursion. When the strong current, the steep mountain pass, or the headwind we face is received as a gift, as an expression of a powerful spirit, our ability to align and move along with it is greatly enhanced. Enlightenment is simply a moment when we experience divinity through the actions of our body and mind; it is a moment when we are in total harmony with the beauty of the world around us.

· HOW TO USE THIS BOOK ·

The first section of this book describes and illustrates twenty-six yoga positions organized in a sequence to reach all major muscle groups while requiring minimal body movement as you progress from one position to the next—certainly an asset when you are performing these routines inside a tent. If the weather is chilly, most poses are possible inside your warm and cozy sleeping bag, although it does require some twisting and scrunching. These positions can be executed just as well on top of your sleeping bag, and inside or outside your tent.

The icons used identify specific positions as being especially beneficial to hikers 𝑋, paddlers 𝘢, or cyclists 𝕕. The accompanying illustrations show the position to work toward. To enhance your overall experience, each position offers either a yoga tip to help you align more effectively, a practical sleeping bag tip, or a Sanskrit term and accompanying meditation.

Ending a day of vigorous exercise by executing the positions in the order they appear in the book will take your body to a relaxed state. In the morning, start from the back of the sequence and work your way forward to energize yourself. The most important guideline, however, is to do what your body and spirit is asking for; I believe our bodies know instinctively what's right for us. Feel free to pick and choose the positions that seem right for a given day.

The second section of the book offers a separate group of positions called the Strengthening Series. These exercises require more space than is available in a tent and more consciousness of your body's limitations. Building strength and endurance is easier and more effective when the body is in proper alignment (any cyclist who has ridden an ill-fitting bike knows the cost of misalignment—ouch!). The series emphasizes proper body alignment as a key to strengthening the core of the body, for when your spine is strengthened while in its natural curvature, harmony is created and you have more endurance. In a kayak, for example, the arms may hold the paddle, but it's core body strength that carries much of the work.

Here are some basic guidelines to help you develop your sleeping bag yoga practice. Refer back to these often to ensure you receive the full benefits of each pose. This book only provides limited instruction; it is best used as a complement to instruction from a skilled teacher, especially if you suffer from injury or chronic pain.

* First, take a moment to soften, and enjoy your surroundings; use a full inhalation to expand and brighten your body.

* Always notice which part of your body is in contact with the earth; be mindful and deliberate in that connection.

- Move with awareness, flowing with the natural pulsation of your breath.

- Fully engage your muscles to the bones, increasing the energetic pull toward the core of your body.

- Tune into your innate wisdom, being conscious of your body's limitations.

- To help bring the hip and shoulder joints into their most protected and optimal alignment, always press the tops of your thighs back and apart and move the tops of the arm bones up and toward the back plane of the body.

- To increase your core strength and help lengthen your lower back, scoop your tailbone by drawing it downward and toning your belly in and up.

- To increase your ability to release tension without diminishing your strength, keep a strong engagement of muscles as you extend your energy and awareness out from the core of your body to its periphery.

- Stay in each position for ten slow breaths, unless there is pain, focusing your attention on the specific muscles you have used throughout the day.

- Keep your facial muscles relaxed and soft, maintaining a soft gaze, as if looking at the most serene of landscapes.

There is nothing quite as exhilarating as traveling under your own power across a beautiful landscape. Practicing *Sleeping Bag Yoga* can enhance your body's health, balance, and strength so that you can fully enjoy each mountain pass, coastal strip, and country road.

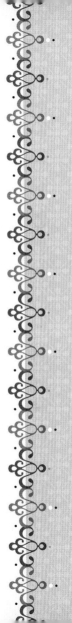

·• twilight position •·

1. Sit comfortably with legs crossed, pelvis and spine fully vertical.

2. Using your breath, extend spine upward, lengthening the sides of your waist and lifting the lowest part of your back in and up to create the natural curve of the spine.

3. Inhale and exhale slowly, expanding lungs and rib cage in all directions as you breathe into every cell. Heighten your awareness to the momentary spaces between the breaths.

Sankalpa: intention

Mindfully setting an intention at the beginning of your practice enhances the will to attain your heart's deepest desire.

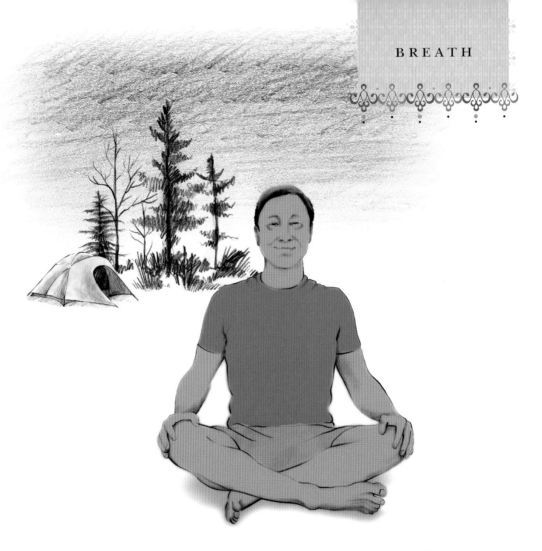

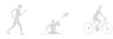

•• moonlight position ••

1. Sit on or between heels, with thighs parallel and toes pointing straight back from the center of your heels. Bring your fingertips to the back of your skull, elbows angling forward and armpits hollow.

2. Press your tailbone down to keep your lower back long; with your breath, lift your whole rib cage upward.

3. Press your head gently into your fingertips, opening your throat as you engage the muscles in your neck and chest to create the natural curve of the cervical spine. Be sure not to overarch the back of the neck.

YOGA TIP: Place a folded-up sleeping bag under your sitbones for support. The back of your pelvis should be vertical, and a natural curve present in your lower back.

● ● ●

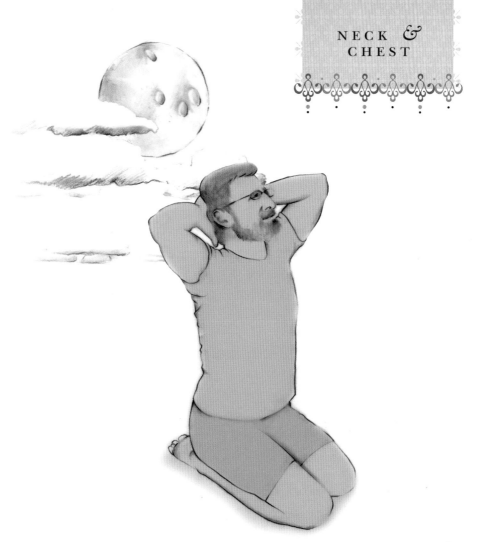

·· ocean swell position ··

1. From Moonlight Position, shift forward, placing your palms on the ground directly beneath your shoulders, fingers spread, with knees directly under hips.

2. Keep your arms straight and strong, and soften your heart and chest toward the floor while breathing into the back of your body.

3. As you inhale, lift your sitbones upward and sweep your heart and gaze forward.

4. As you exhale, scoop your tailbone down toward the earth to create a lift in the belly, and release the head completely.

5. Move back and forth between positions, feeling each breath travel the entire length of your spine.

Spanda: pulsation

Move with the natural pulsation of life as expressed through the innate action of your body's cells as well as the mighty ocean tides.

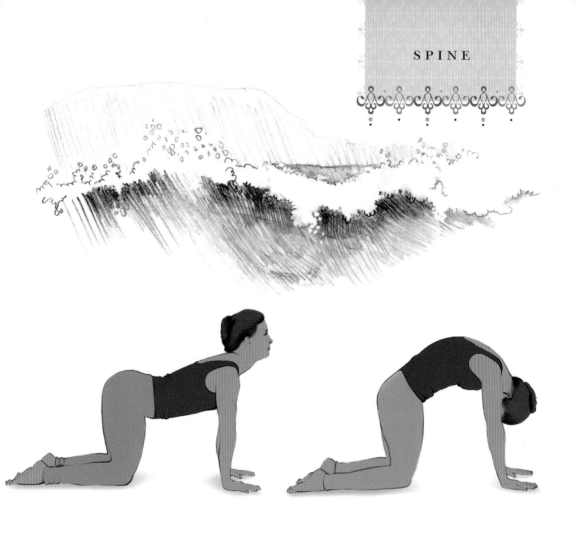

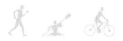

·• root position •·

1. From Ocean Swell Position, tuck toes under, placing balls of feet on the ground; spread your toes.

2. Shift your hips back, resting weight on heels to stretch the soles of your feet.

3. Reach arms forward, pressing your fingertips strongly into the earth; lift the upper arm bones to the sky. Release the center of your heart down to the earth.

YOGA TIP: To help alleviate any knee pain, push an edge of your sleeping bag against the back of your knees, under your thighs, to create space under the knee joint.

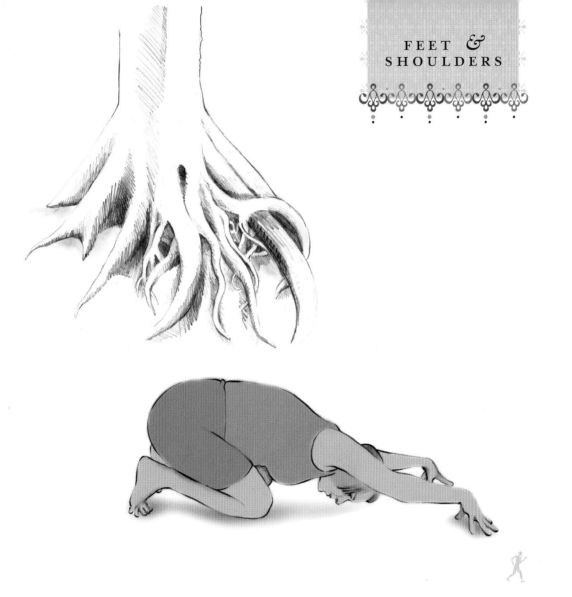

·• mountain pass position •·

1. From Root Position, flatten palms to the earth, move pelvis squarely up and back while keeping feet and knees parallel.

2. Press palms, especially the base of the index finger, strongly into the earth to keep a lift in the arm bones and inner shoulders.

3. Keeping legs parallel, bend your knees and lift your sitbones to their highest peak, then stretch your thighs farther back, straightening the legs and lowering your heels.

Satya: truth

Be true to your greatest ability and potential.

● ● ●

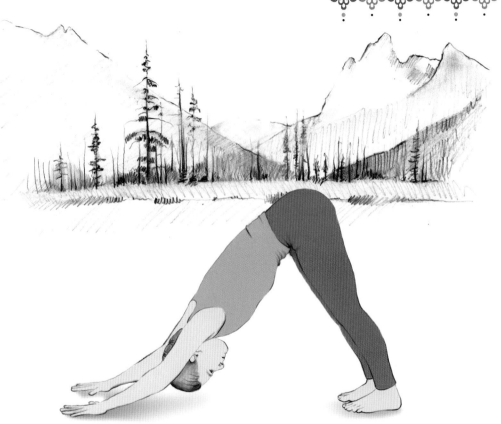

·• crosswind position •·

1. From Mountain Pass Position, press strongly into your right palm all the way out to the tips of your fingers, keeping a stable lift under the right inner shoulder.

2. Lift your left palm and place it on the outside of your right leg.

3. Extend from your heart up the spine and down the legs to hold pelvis and legs stable; use your breath to twist your torso to the right.

4. Repeat with opposite side.

SLEEPING BAG TIP: Using a large stuff sack with compression straps makes packing easier and keeps the carrying size small.

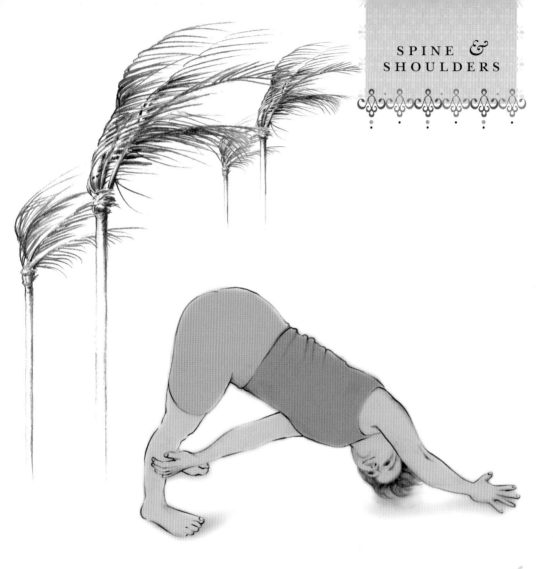

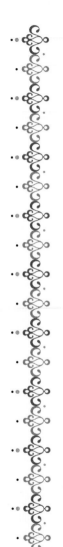

·· riverbank position ··

1. From Mountain Pass Position (page 18), step your feet forward behind your palms, placing feet hip width apart and parallel with each other.

2. Bend your knees a couple of inches; press the balls of your feet strongly into the earth and spread your toes.

3. Lift your sitbones and create a curve in your lower back, heart sweeping forward.

4. Bring your hands to the outside of your shins. Keeping knees ankle width apart, press your hands toward each other and actively widen your inner thighs.

Anugraha: grace
Flow with a movement toward beauty.

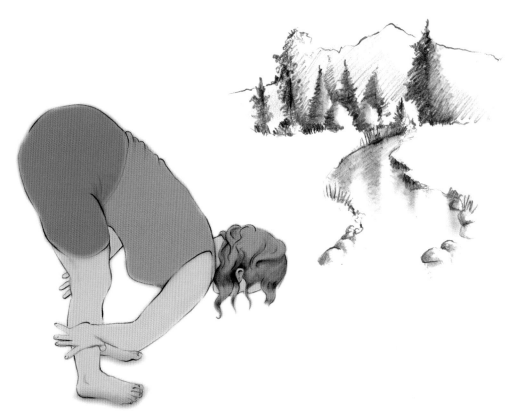

·· undercurrent position ··

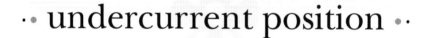

1. From Riverbank Position, shift your weight to your left foot and cross your right ankle over the base of your left thigh. Either keep the right hand on the earth or hold the right knee.

2. Keeping your right foot flexed, move your pinky toe toward your knee, and press the ball of your big toe into your left hand.

3. Allow a deep current of opening to occur in your hip joints.

4. Repeat with opposite side.

SLEEPING BAG TIP: Placing the sleeping bag up high in the front compartment of your kayak keeps the bow light, easing your glide through the water.

HIPS

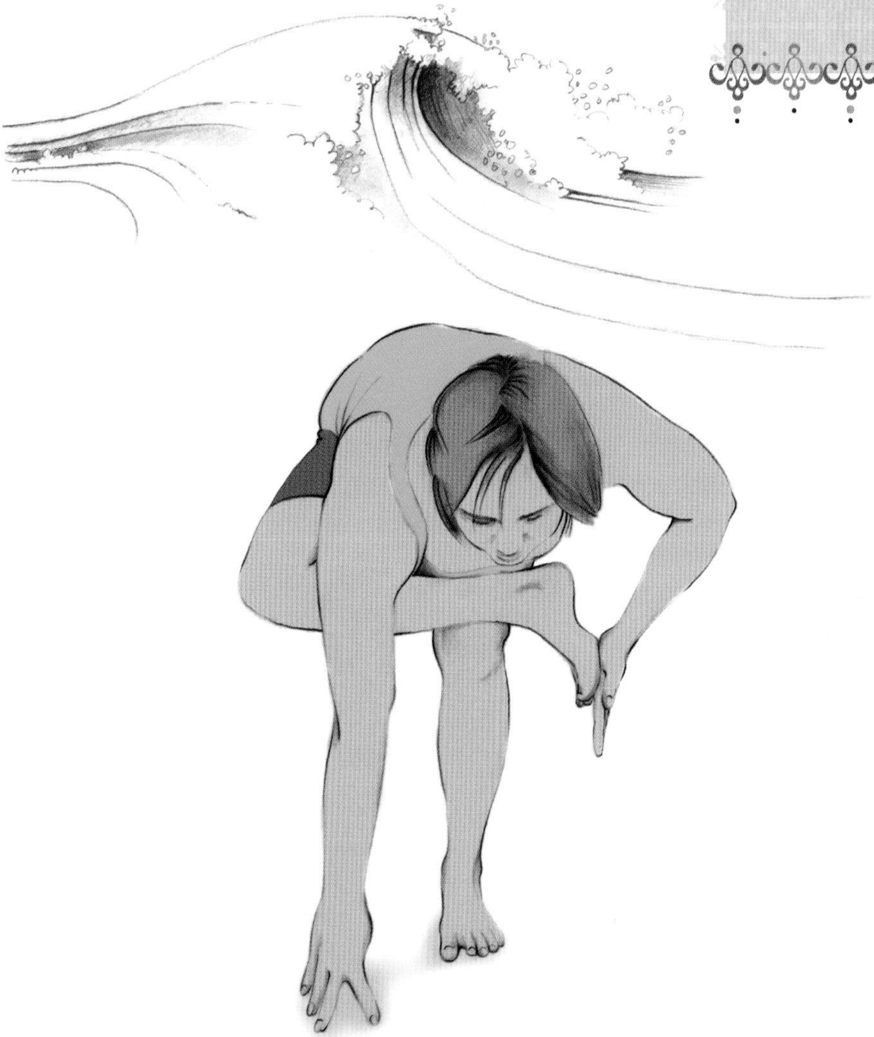

·· thundercloud position ··

1. From Riverbank Position (page 22), widen feet to outer hip width apart, sitbones still lifting to the sky. Slowly bend knees fully, turning knees and feet out if necessary.

2. Bring your palms together in front of your heart. Hug your knees against your upper arm bones as you press your arms out into your knees.

3. Keep the balls of your big toes rooted into the earth as you extend your spine upward, lengthening the sides of your waist.

4. Let the weight of your pelvis descend as you actively open your heart and smile to the sky above.

YOGA TIP: Fold the sleeping bag and place under heels for more support.

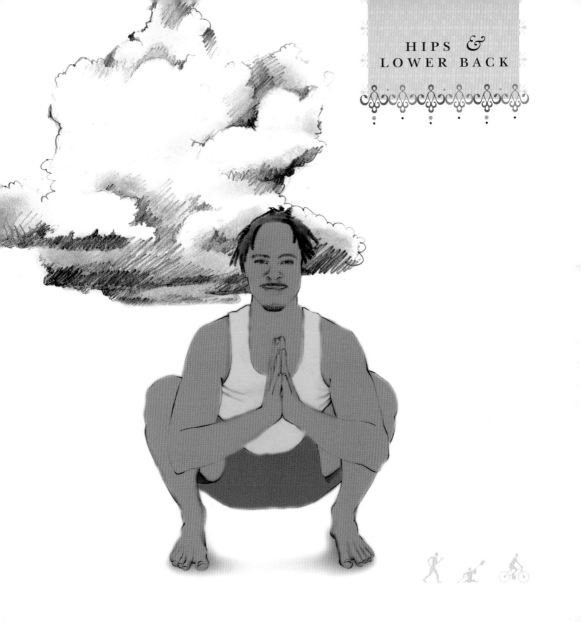

·• overhang position •·

1. From Thundercloud Position, place your hands on the earth shoulder distance apart with fingers spread wide and upper arm bones pressing into your shins.

2. Hug your legs into your arms as you shift your weight forward, bringing elbows right over your wrists. Look forward and lift your spreading toes off the ground.

3. From your heart, press your hands and fingers down and lift your lower back to the sky.

Adbhuta: wonder

Open your eyes and heart to the mystery of the world.

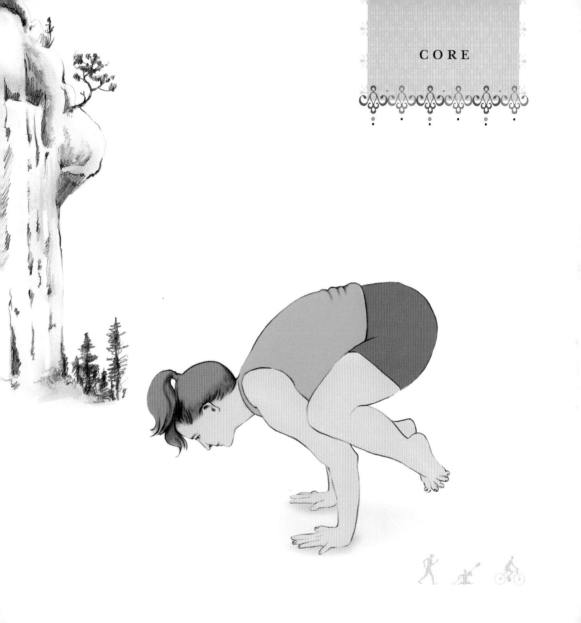

·• new growth position •·

1. Lay on your belly with toes pointing straight back behind you and tops of feet pressing into the earth.

2. Extend your arms back behind you, interlacing your fingers, with elbows slightly bent.

3. Scoop your tailbone, lengthen the sides of your waist, and move your whole rib cage forward. Inhale and sweep the heart forward and up, raising your upper arm bones.

4. Draw your shoulder blades deeply into the back as you extend the crown of your head toward the sky, keeping the back of the neck long.

SLEEPING BAG TIP: Using a plastic bag inside of the stuff sack keeps the bag dry during any weather conditions and protects the plastic from tearing.

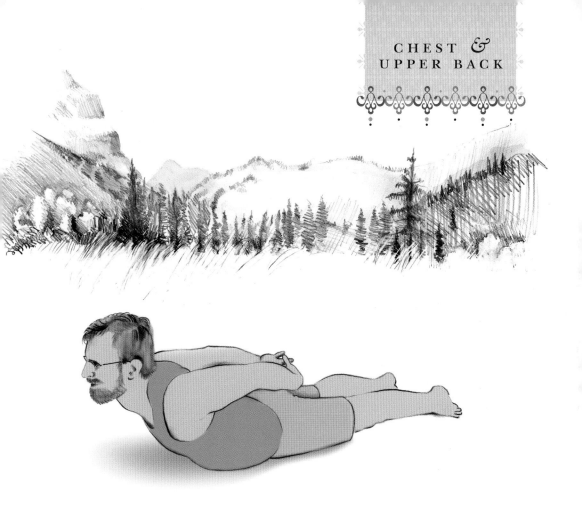

·• many miles position •·

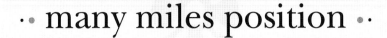

1. From New Growth Position, bring your left forearm to cross in front of your chest. Bend your right leg, keeping knee pressed into the earth. Reach back with right hand to hold top of foot, scooping the tailbone strongly to the earth.

2. Press foot strongly into hand, spreading toes. Sweep your chest forward, right shoulder drawing back and neck long.

3. Extend from your pelvis out through the bent leg as you bend right elbow to bring foot closer to the outside of your hip.

4. Repeat with opposite side.

Svatantrya: freedom

Express your innate freedom by choosing actions that honor the beauty of the world around you.

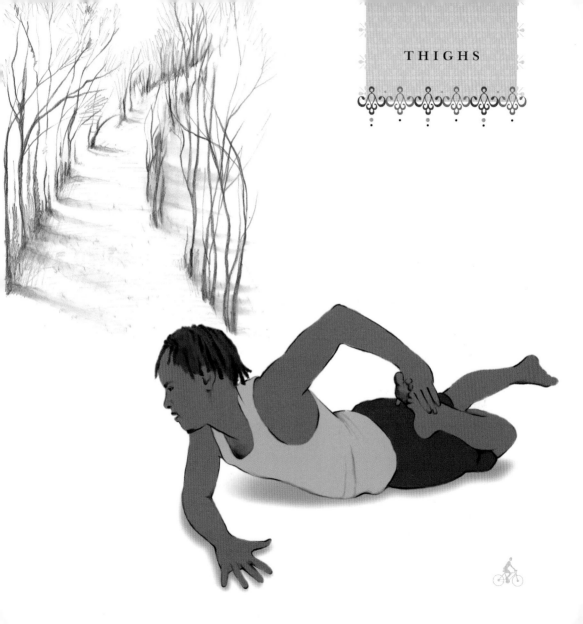

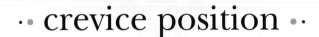

·• crevice position •·

1. Sit with feet on the ground, knees bent. Inhale and bring arms straight out in front of your shoulders. Expand the chest and bring the upper arm bones deep into the back of the shoulder sockets, palms facing each other.

2. Lean your torso back as you lift your chest and legs toward the sky, spreading your toes.

3. Straighten your legs only as far as you can keep your chest lifted.

Daksina: gift

Express your gratitude: move through your environment by leaving it cleaner than when you arrived.

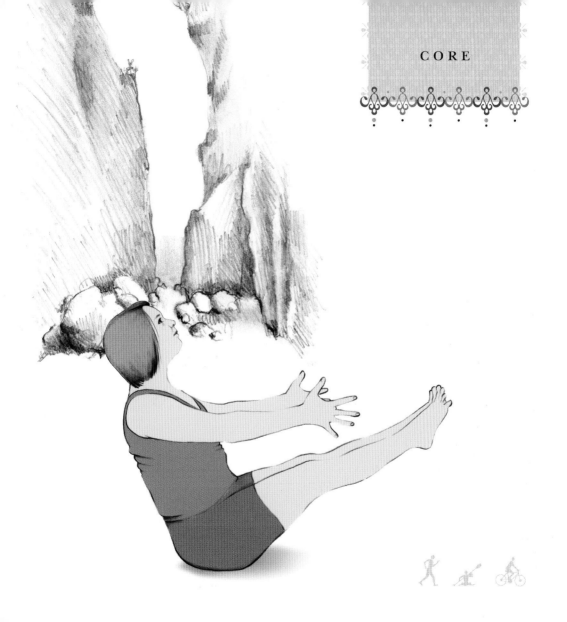

· headwind position ··

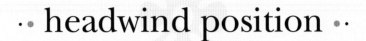

1. From Mountain Pass Position (page 18), bring right foot forward, bending the knee right over your front heel; place your fingertips on either side of your front foot.

2. Lift your back thigh straight and strong away from the earth while pressing the front foot firmly into the earth.

3. Keep the pelvis square to the front as you extend out through the back heel and the front knee simultaneously.

4. Repeat with opposite side.

SLEEPING BAG TIP: Placing your sleeping bag on top of the back rack while cycle touring allows for more room in the panniers without affecting wind resistance.

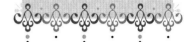

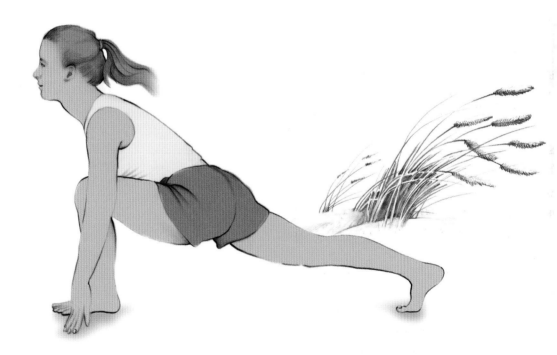

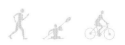

·• whirlpool position •·

1. Sit with legs straight out in front and feet flexed. Bend right knee, placing foot firmly on the ground, as if to stand.

2. Inhale and draw lower back in and up, lifting the chest and expanding the side body and spine into its fullest extension.

3. Keeping your pelvis steady, on your exhale, start with the lower back, moving up toward your neck and skull, spiral each vertebra as far around its axis as your breath allows. Use your left hand on your knee to support the extension in your spine.

4. Repeat on opposite side.

YOGA TIP: Sit on a folded-up sleeping bag for height; the back of your pelvis should be vertical, and a natural curve present in your lower back.

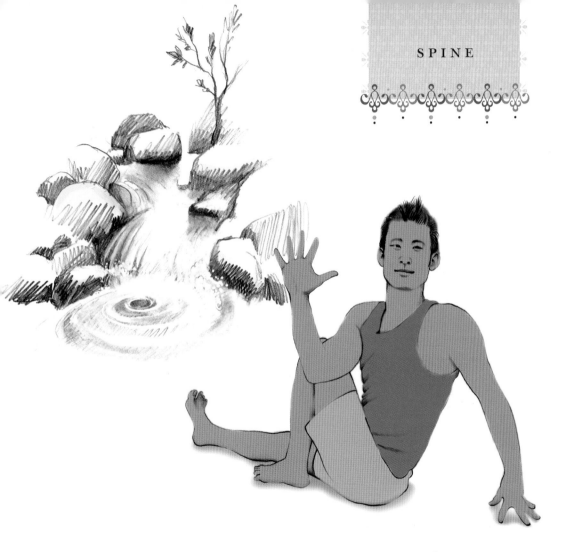

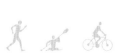

·• sunrise position ·•

1. From Whirlpool Position, open right knee out at an angle. Bring the heel of the right foot into the right inner thigh, while keeping the left knee and toes facing straight upward. Press the top of the right foot strongly into the earth, both sitbones grounded.

2. Lengthen both sides of the waist and slide the left hand along the inside of the left leg, potentially holding the big toe; bring the left arm in line with your ear.

3. Keeping your pelvis steady, rotate the front torso upward and lift the right shoulder up and back. Use your elbow or palm against the inside of your leg for added support. Use each exhalation to move deeper into the twist.

4. Repeat with opposite side.

Hasya: lightheartedness
Be light with the rising sun; laugh with the joy of a new day.

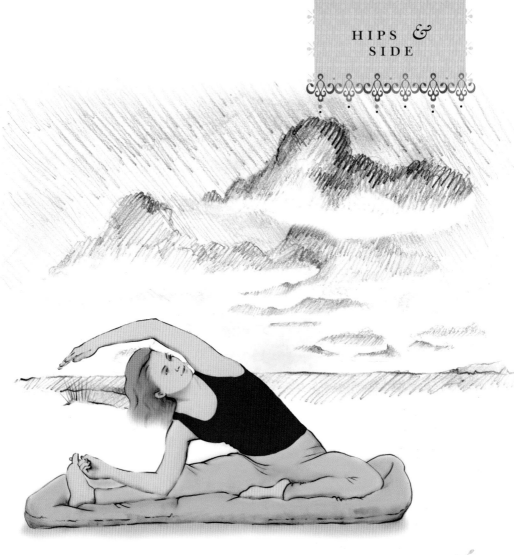

·• sunset position •·

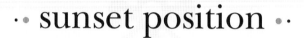

1. From Sunrise Position, bring your hands beside your pelvis for support and rotate the front of your torso to face the straightened leg.

2. Inhale and tilt your upper pelvis forward, lengthening both sides of your body and widening the sitbones.

3. Scoop your tailbone toward the earth, and extend your chest toward your shins. With each exhalation soften and descend deeper into the stretch.

4. Repeat with opposite side.

Namaste: to bow

Bow and be humble in the magnificence of your surroundings.

● ● ●

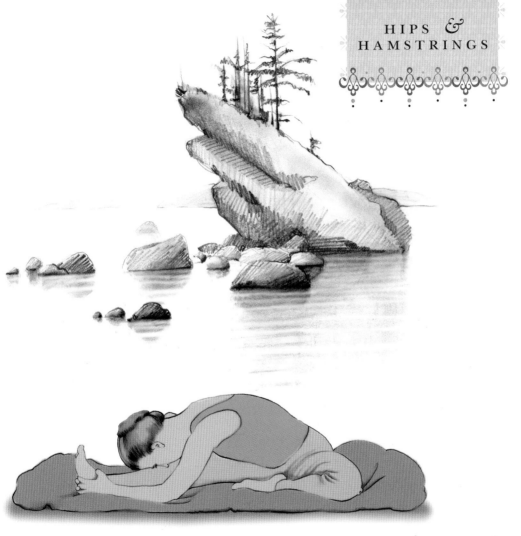

·• river rock position •·

1. From Sunset Position, straighten both legs out in front of you with pelvis vertical and a natural curve present in your lower back, press through balls of your feet, spreading your toes.

2. Inhale and tilt your upper pelvis forward, widening the sitbones.

3. Scoop your tailbone toward the earth, and extend your chest toward your shins.

4. Expand with the motion of your breath. With each inhalation, extend the spine toward your toes; with each exhalation, release your chest toward your shins.

YOGA TIP: Sit on a folded-up sleeping bag for height; the back of your pelvis should start out vertical with a natural curve present in your lower back.

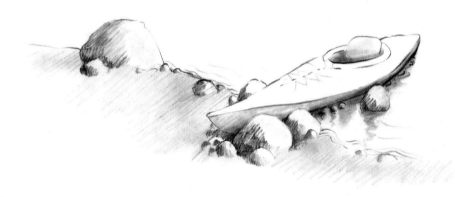

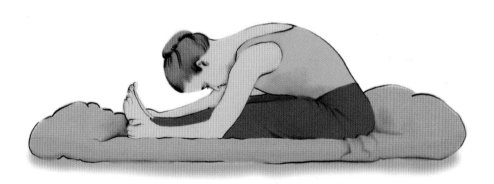

·· burning log position ··

1. From River Rock Position, sit with pelvis upright and sitbones wide. Place your outer left shin on the earth in front of you with foot strongly flexed. Keeping foot flexed, place right shin on top of left, ankle directly on top of knee.

2. Bring your hands onto balls of feet; press strongly through ball of big toe to create length in the inner ankle and protect your knee while expanding back of pelvis.

3. Keeping spine long, fold forward.

4. Repeat with opposite side.

YOGA TIP: Move feet farther away from pelvis and place ankles on top of each other if position is difficult to create, or place sleeping bag under outer ankle of top leg for support.

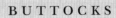
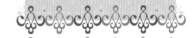
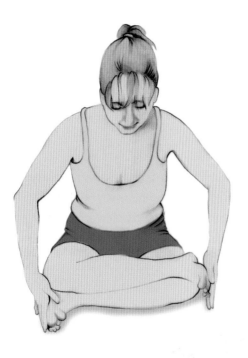

·• lightning bolt position •·

1. From Burning Log Position, lie back, placing feet wide apart yet parallel. Bring your upper arms alongside your ribs, pointing fingertips up to the sky.

2. Gently press back of head, upper arm bones, and sitbones into the earth to open throat and create a curve in lower back.

3. Lower your right knee toward your left foot, pressing the inside edge of the flexed foot into the earth.

4. Repeat with opposite side.

SLEEPING BAG TIP: **Placing your sleeping bag as low as you can in your backpack provides better hip padding and weight distribution.**

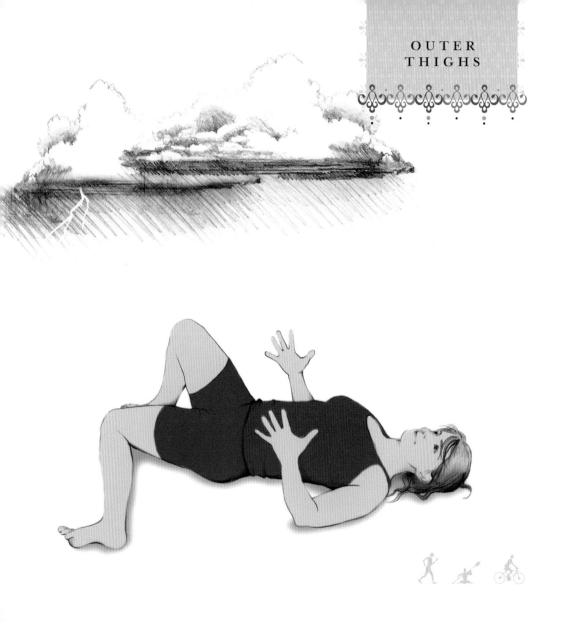

·• arches position •··

1. From Lightning Bolt Position, bring feet back to hip width apart and parallel. Keep pressing back of head, upper arm bones, and sitbones into the earth to open throat and create a curve in lower back.

2. Press your parallel feet into the earth, inhale, and lift your pelvis up toward the sky.

3. Without locking your elbows, interlace your fingers under pelvis. Press upper arms downward, rolling shoulders open and back, without drawing them away from your ears.

4. Inhale fully, expanding the chest and extending the spine into an arch.

YOGA TIP: **Place your stuffed sleeping bag between your knees and squeeze strongly to help alleviate any lower back pain.**

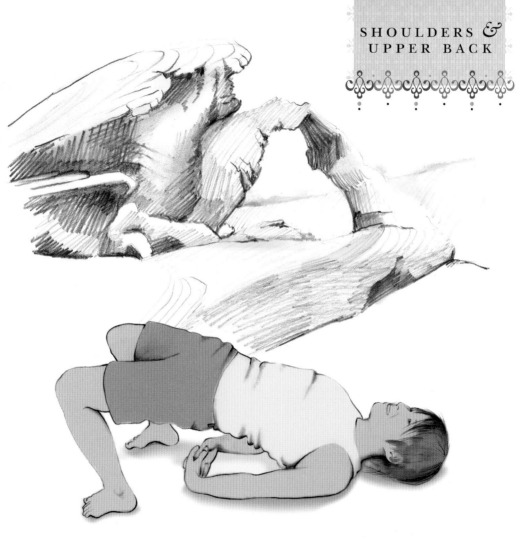

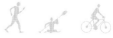

·• canyon wall position •·

1. From Arches Position, bring sit-bones back to ground, keeping a slight arch in the lower back. Extend your left leg flat against the earth, pressing through the ball of the foot with toes pointing to the sky.

2. Keep your left thigh pressing down, draw your right knee toward your chest, and interlace your fingers behind your thigh.

3. Press your thigh strongly into your hands, away from your chest, to release the muscles attached to the vertebrae of your lower back. Extend through both feet.

4. Repeat on opposite side.

Sukha: ease

Delight in your body's innate wisdom and intelligent design.

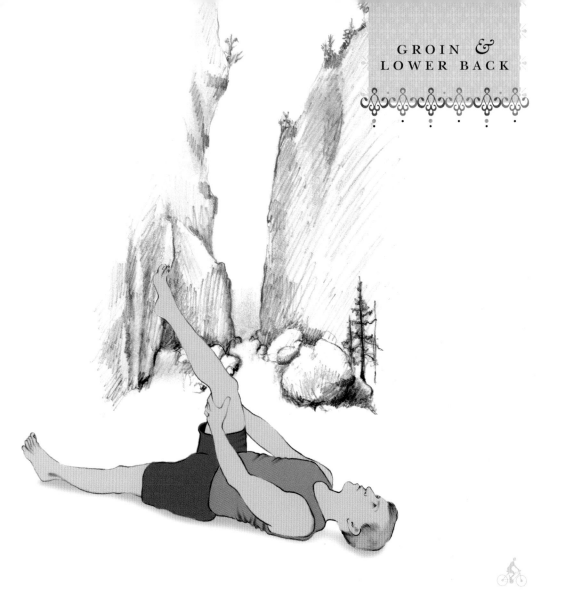

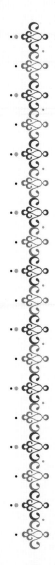

·• switchback position •·

1. From Canyon Wall Position, bend left knee and place right flexed foot on left thigh. Interlace hands around back of left thigh.

2. Keep pressing the back of thigh into your hands as you push angled right knee away from body.

3. Repeat with opposite side.

 SLEEPING BAG TIP: Between trips, store your sleeping bag uncompressed to help preserve its loft.

● ● ●

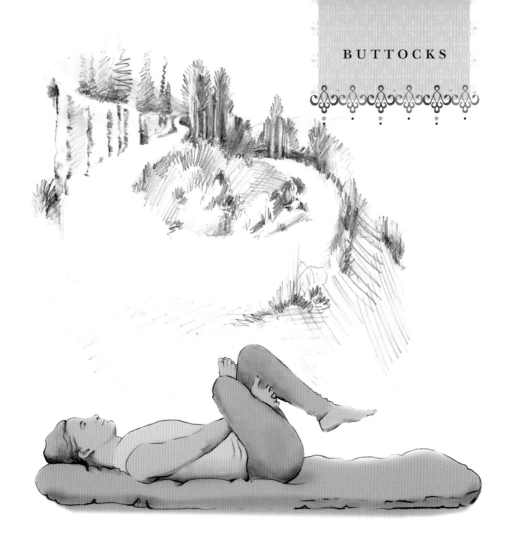

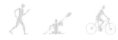

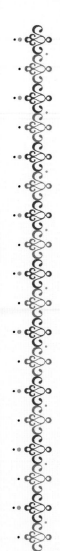

·· fallen log position ··

1. From Switchback Position, bring legs together, thighs vertical. Stretch arms out to either side at shoulder height, with palms facing down for stability.

2. Keeping a slight curve in the back and your right shoulder heavy on the ground, rotate knees to left.

3. Use smooth, deep breathing to release tension in lower spine.

4. Repeat with opposite side.

Ananda: bliss

The nature of the world offers itself as a gift to you; delight in it.

● ● ●

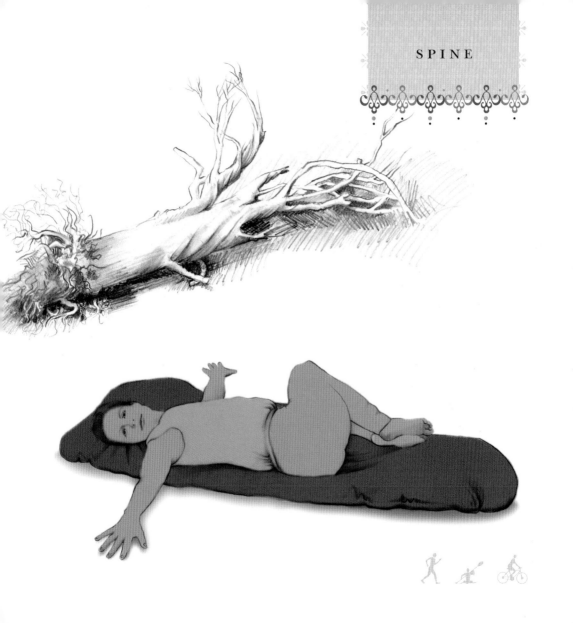

·· hibernation position ··

1. Come to a hands and knees position, widen your knees, and touch your toes back behind you. Shift your pelvis back onto your heels.

2. Stretch arms forward, bringing your forearms and forehead to the earth. Gently use the weight of your head to draw the skin on your forehead toward your eyebrows.

3. Relax your spine, softening any muscular tension and slowing down your body processes by focusing on your breathing.

YOGA TIP: Rest your head on a sleeping bag or place an edge of the bag behind your knees under your thighs for additional support.

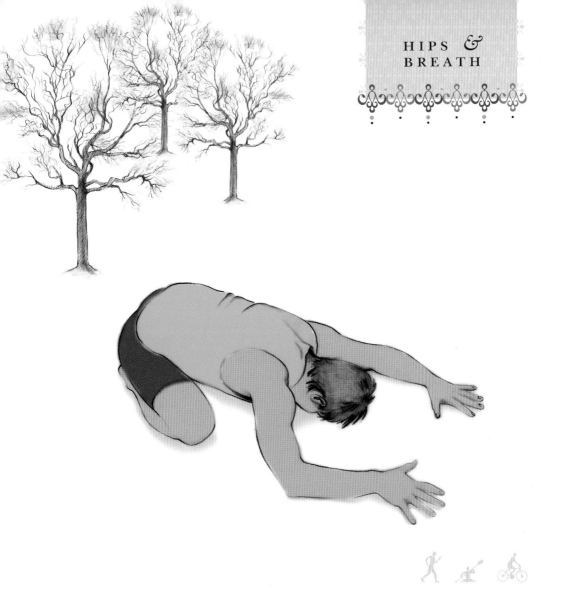

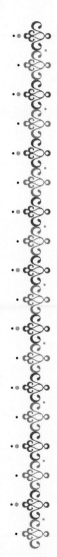

·• reflection position ••

1. Lie flat on your back with arm and leg muscles completely released.

2. Allow your body to absorb the oxygen you have circulated throughout your muscles and joints, just as the mountain lake absorbs the reflection of the mountain that feeds it.

Shanti: peace

Be still and smile.

● ● ●

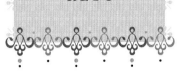

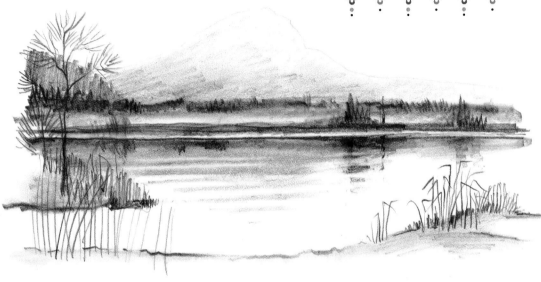

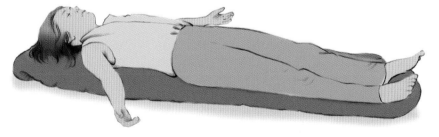

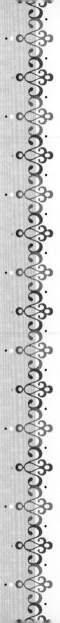

·• strengthening series •·

OF TWELVE POSES

As you take that inevitable break between miles, practice the following Strengthening Series to rejuvenate your mind and body. This sequence will actually release tension in overworked muscles, realign your spine, and prepare your muscles for further use. Over time, it will strengthen the core body muscles you need to perform sports efficiently. This sequence can also shift the flow of your mind back into the spirit of play, and harmonize your heart to pulse more freely with the vibrancy of life.

❊   The series describes a strengthening sequence of twelve positions. To complete a basic sequence, begin with number one and move through the twelve positions, doing both sides for positions number five through eight, then step forward to create the beginning of number four and work backward to number one. You will end in the position in which you began, ready for an additional sequence.

❋ This series includes more challenging positions; please refer back to the initial guidelines on page 7 to assist in creating the safest and most optimal practice.

❋ As you practice the Strengthening Series, move smoothly from one position to the next, following your breath cycle.

Shri: abundance, value, benevolence

In the beauty of the light, revel in all that's around you, for it simply reflects the sweetness that resides inside you.

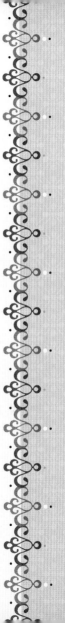

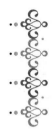

POSE NO.
01

STAND WITH YOUR FEET HIP DISTANCE APART and parallel with each other. Touching palms together in front of your heart, breathe fully and expand the sides of your body and spine directly upward.

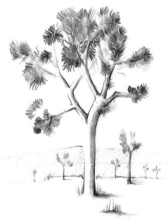

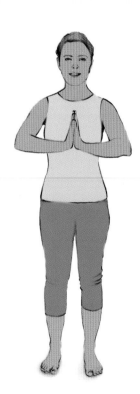

INHALE AND SWEEP YOUR ARMS UP and overhead in line with ears. Keeping thighs back and legs strong, begin lifting chest and arching upper back.

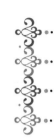

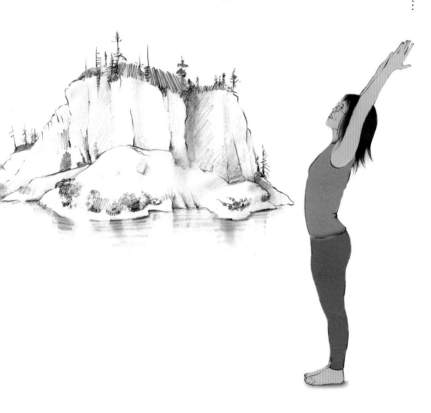

POSE NO.

03

EXHALE AND FOLD FORWARD leading with your heart, touch fingertips to the earth or, if needed, your shins. Keeping legs straight, lift sitbones up and release your heart and torso fully.

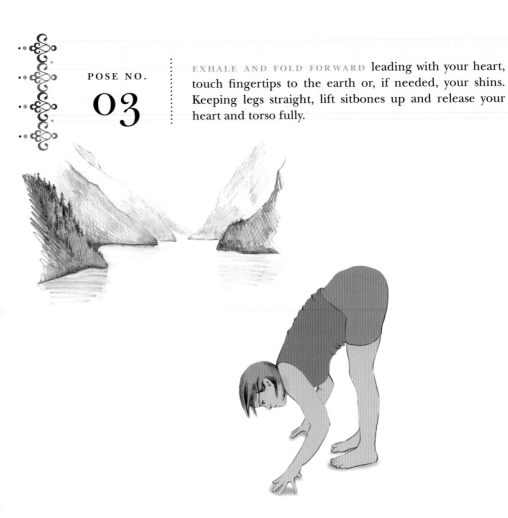

PRESS THE BALLS OF YOUR FEET strongly into the earth and bend your knees. Scoop your tailbone and move your waistline back to bring your torso upright. Inhale and sweep your arms in line with your ears.

POSE NO.

04

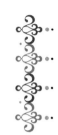

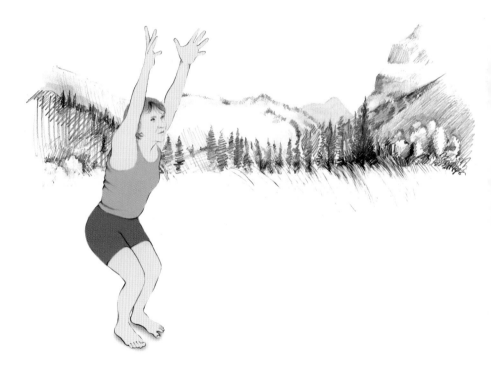

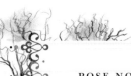

POSE NO.

05

BRING YOUR FINGERTIPS TO PRESS strongly into the earth on either side of feet. Reach one foot back behind you while bending the opposite leg into a lunge; keep your pelvis square to the front as you extend your back leg straight.

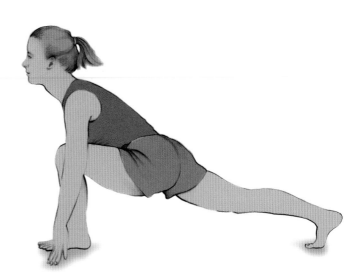

HOLD YOUR PELVIS AND LEGS STEADY; rotate your belly, torso, and shoulder toward the bent leg as you lift your arm to the sky.

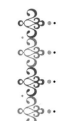

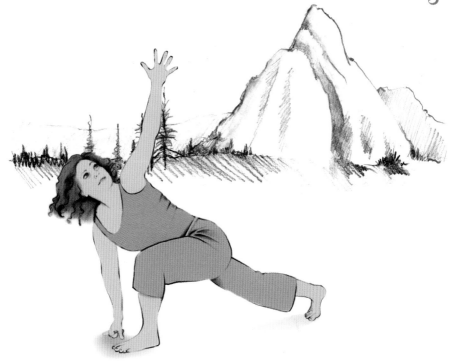

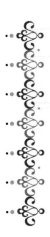

BRING ALL TEN FINGERTIPS BACK TO THE EARTH.
Pivot your back heel to the earth perpendicular to the
front foot and fully straighten the back leg, pressing the
top of the back thigh bone back a couple of inches to align
the hip joints. Keeping the feet strongly pressed into the
earth, scoop your tailbone to open your pelvis, belly, and
shoulders away from the front leg. Lengthen both sides
of your waist as you sweep your arm in line with your ear,
palm facedown. If needed, slide elbow up to press onto
the thigh.

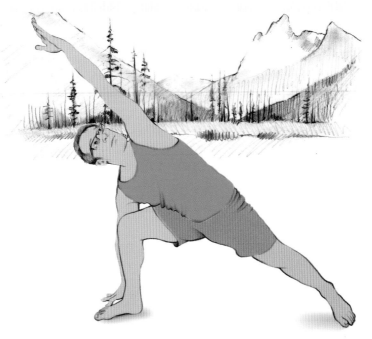

KEER YOUR FEET PRESSING INTO THE EARTH and straighten your front leg fully. Pivot top arm to extend fully upright and lean your head and top shoulder back.

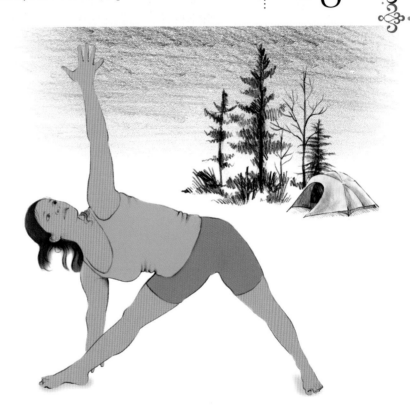

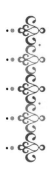

POSE NO.

09

BRING PALMS BACK TO THE EARTH and slide front leg to join back leg, with feet hip width apart. Have your shoulders right over your wrists with creases of the wrists straight across, fingers spread. From your pelvis, extend out through heels and crown of head, keeping whole body on the same plane.

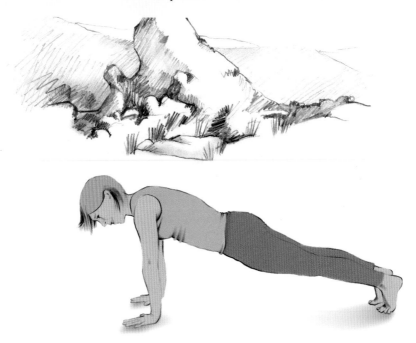

BEND YOUR ELBOWS TO BRING SHOULDERS to elbow height, keeping shoulder blades strong on the back and your head in line with the spine.

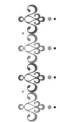

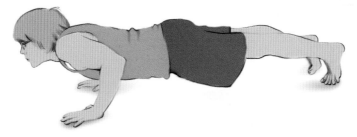

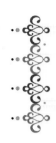

POSE NO.

11

WITHOUT DROPPING SHOULDERS, release your pelvis to the earth and come to the tops of your feet. Press toenails, tailbone, and palms down as you sweep your heart forward and lift shoulders up and back, neck long.

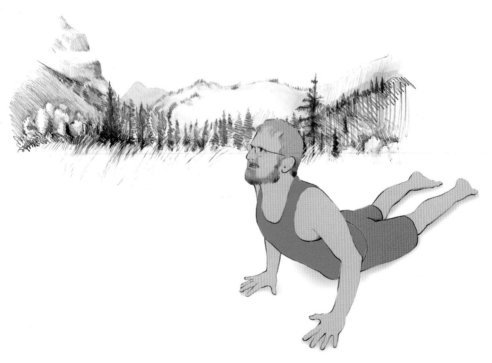

PRESS YOUR PALMS AND FINGERS strongly into the earth and lift your pelvis up and back, straightening the legs and bringing the heels toward the earth.

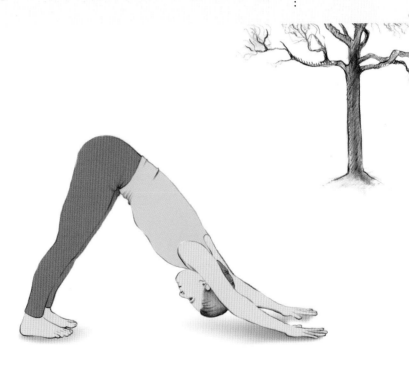

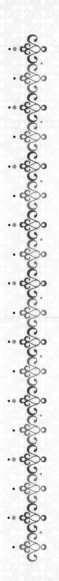

·· appendix ··

The poses in this book will look familiar to anyone who has practiced yoga, as many of them are done in any Hatha yoga practice. This book offers a new set of names for the poses simply to give the practitioner a qualitative or poetic feel for the pose. For those who are interested, here is a listing of both the Sanskrit and common Western name for each pose described.

Positions

POSE NAME	SANSKRIT NAME	COMMON WESTERN NAME
Twilight	*Sukhasana*	Easy Seat Pose
Moonlight	*Virasana* (variation)	Hero Pose
Ocean Swell	(varies)	Cow and Cat Pose
Root	*Utthita Balasana*	Extended Child's Pose
Mountain Pass	*Adho Mukha Svanasana*	Downward Facing Dog
Crosswind	*Parivrtta Adho Mukha Svanasana*	Revolved Downward Facing Dog
Riverbank*	*Uttanasana* (variation)	Standing Forward Bend

POSE NAME	SANSKRIT NAME	COMMON WESTERN NAME
Undercurrent*	*Ardha Baddha Padmottanasana*	Standing Half-Bound Lotus Pose
Thundercloud	*Malasana*	Garland Pose, Squat
Overhang	*Bakasana*	Crane Pose
New Growth*	*Salabhasana*	Locust Pose
Many Miles	*Ardha Bhekasana*	Half Frog Pose
Crevice	*Navasana*	Boat Pose
Headwind*	*Virabhadrasana I*	Lunge Pose
Whirlpool	*Marichyasana III*	Seated Twist
Sunrise	*Parivrtta Janu Sirsasana*	Revolved Head to Knee
Sunset	*Janu Sirsasana*	Head to Knee
River Rock	*Paschimottanasana*	Seated Forward Bend
Burning Log	*Agnistambhasana*	Burning Log Pose
Lightning Bolt	*Vayu Kavicha Shuddhi Krtasana*	Windshield Wiper Pose
Arches	*Setu Bandha Sarvangasana*	Bridge Pose
Canyon Wall*	*Supta Padangusthasana*	Reclined Hand to Big Toe
Switchback	*Sucirandhrasana*	Eye of the Needle
Fallen Log*	*Jathara Parivartanasana*	Revolved Belly Pose
Hibernation	*Pranam*	Extended Child's Pose
Reflection	*Savasana*	Corpse Pose

*Indicates pose is a preparation for the full pose.

Strengthening Series

POSE NO.	SANSKRIT NAME	COMMON WESTERN NAME
01	*Tadasana*	Mountain Pose
02	*Urdhva Tadasana*	Upward Facing Mountain Pose
03	*Uttanasana*	Standing Forward Bend
04	*Utkatasana*	Fierce Pose
05	*Virabhadrasana I**	Lunge Pose
06	*Parivrrta Parsvakonasana**	Revolved Side Angle Pose
07	*Utthita Parsvakonasana*	Extended Side Angle Pose
08	*Trikonasana*	Triangle Pose
09	*Talakasana*	Plank Pose
10	*Chaturanga Dandasana*	Four-Limbed Staff Pose
11	*Bhujangasana*	Cobra Pose
12	*Adho Mukha Svanasana*	Downward Facing Dog

*Indicates pose is a preparation for the full pose.

·• about the author ·•

Erin Widman is an Anusara-inspired Yoga Teacher™ in Flagstaff, Arizona, where she is owner and director of The Yoga Experience (www.theyogaexperience .com). She spent a decade as an outdoor educator and has traveled throughout the United States, India, Nepal, New Zealand, Bolivia, and Peru. She currently spends her time traveling through the vast landscape of motherhood with her two delightful children, who now educate her on the wonders of the outdoors.

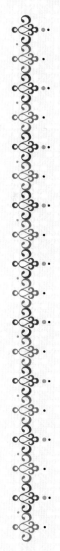